There is a saying – you can't

manage

what you don't measure.

Measuring your intake helps you

manage your output.

A healthier inside makes for a

more attractive outside.

Become your own Boss
today, by managing what
you eat, and how you use
those calories

Notes:

Mahatma Gandhi

Your beliefs become your
thoughts,
Your thoughts become
your words,
Your words become your
actions,
**Your actions become
your habits,**
**Your habits become your
values,**
Your values become your
destiny.

Notes:

Becoming aware of your actions helps to make sure you are taking the right ones.

www.hiddenvalleypress.com/shop

Negative Habit	Why is it a negative habit?	What steps can I take to change it?

Notes:

Habit Tracker

Month _____

Year _____

Day														
1														
2														
3														
4														
5														
6														
7														
8														
9														
10														
11														
12														
13														
14														
15														
16														
17														
18														
19														
20														
21														
22														
23														
24														
25														
26														
27														
28														
29														
30														
31														

Notes:

Don't let what you didn't do today get in the way of you can do tomorrow!

Date:

6 am	
7	
8	
9	
10	
11	
12 pm	
1	
2	
3	
4	
5	
6	
7	
8	

To Do

Happiness

100%

75%   45%

60%

Accomplishments

☐ . . . .

☐ . . . .

☐ . . . .

☐ . . . .

Notes:_____

_____

_____

_____

Date		S M T W T F S	
Breakfast		Amount	Calories (kcal)
		Total	
Snack		Amount	Calories (kcal)
		Total	
Lunch		Amount	Calories (kcal)
		Total	

Snack	Amount	Calories (kcal)
	Total	
Dinner	Amount	Calories (kcal)
	Total	
Snack	Amount	Calories (kcal)
	Total	
Exercise	Duration	Calories burned (kcal)

Water									Fruit & Veggies								

Notes:

Don't rush the process, consistence delivers results!

Date:

6 am	
7	
8	
9	
10	
11	
12 pm	
1	
2	
3	
4	
5	
6	
7	
8	

To Do

Happiness

100%

75%   45%

60%

Accomplishments

☐. . . . .
☐. . . . .
☐. . . . .
☐. . . . .

Notes:_____
_____
_____
_____

Date		S M T W T F S	
Breakfast		Amount	Calories (kcal)
		Total	
Snack		Amount	Calories (kcal)
		Total	
Lunch		Amount	Calories (kcal)
		Total	

Snack	Amount	Calories (kcal)
	Total	
Dinner	Amount	Calories (kcal)
	Total	
Snack	Amount	Calories (kcal)
	Total	
Exercise	Duration	Calories burned (kcal)

Water									Fruit & Veggies								

Notes:

Don't let what you didn't do today get in the way of you can do tomorrow!

Date:

6 am	
7	
8	
9	
10	
11	
12 pm	
1	
2	
3	
4	
5	
6	
7	
8	

Notes: _____
_____
_____
_____

To Do

Happiness

100%

75%   45%

60%

Accomplishments

☐ . . . .
☐ . . . .
☐ . . . .
☐ . . . .

Date	S M T W T F S	
Breakfast	Amount	Calories (kcal)
	Total	
Snack	Amount	Calories (kcal)
	Total	
Lunch	Amount	Calories (kcal)
	Total	

Snack	Amount	Calories (kcal)
	Total	
Dinner	Amount	Calories (kcal)
	Total	
Snack	Amount	Calories (kcal)
	Total	
Exercise	Duration	Calories burned (kcal)
Water									Fruit & Veggies								

Notes:

Don't rush the process, consistence delivers results!

Date:

6 am	
7	
8	
9	
10	
11	
12 pm	
1	
2	
3	
4	
5	
6	
7	
8	

To Do

Happiness

100%

75%   45%

60%

Accomplishments

☐ . . . .
☐ . . . .
☐ . . . .
☐ . . . .

Notes:_____

_____

_____

_____

Date	S M T W T F S	
Breakfast	Amount	Calories (kcal)
	Total	
Snack	Amount	Calories (kcal)
	Total	
Lunch	Amount	Calories (kcal)
	Total	

Snack	Amount	Calories (kcal)
	Total	
Dinner	Amount	Calories (kcal)
	Total	
Snack	Amount	Calories (kcal)
	Total	
Exercise	Duration	Calories burned (kcal)

Water									Fruit & Veggies								

Notes:

Don't let what you didn't do today get in the way of you can do tomorrow!

6 am

7

8

9

10

11

12 pm

1

2

3

4

5

6

7

8

Notes:_____

_____

_____

_____

To Do

Happiness

100%

75%   45%

60%

Accomplishments

☐ . . . .

☐ . . . .

☐ . . . .

☐ . . . .

Date		S M T W T F S	
Breakfast		Amount	Calories (kcal)
		Total	
Snack		Amount	Calories (kcal)
		Total	
Lunch		Amount	Calories (kcal)
		Total	

Snack	Amount	Calories (kcal)
	Total	
Dinner	Amount	Calories (kcal)
	Total	
Snack	Amount	Calories (kcal)
	Total	
Exercise	Duration	Calories burned (kcal)

Water									Fruit & Veggies							

Notes:

Don't rush the process, consistence delivers results!

Date:

Time	
6 am	
7	
8	
9	
10	
11	
12 pm	
1	
2	
3	
4	
5	
6	
7	
8	

To Do

Happiness

100%

75%   45%

60%

Accomplishments

☐ . . . .
☐ . . . .
☐ . . . .
☐ . . . .

Notes:_____

_____

_____

_____

Date		S M T W T F S	
Breakfast		Amount	Calories (kcal)
		Total	
Snack		Amount	Calories (kcal)
		Total	
Lunch		Amount	Calories (kcal)
		Total	

Snack	Amount	Calories (kcal)
	Total	
Dinner	Amount	Calories (kcal)
	Total	
Snack	Amount	Calories (kcal)
	Total	
Exercise	Duration	Calories burned (kcal)

Water										Fruit & Veggies							

Notes:

Don't let what you didn't do today get in the way of you can do tomorrow!

Date:

6 am	To Do
7	
8	
9	
10	
11	
12 pm	
1	Happiness
2	
3	100%
4	75% 45%
5	60%
6	
7	Accomplishments
8	

Notes:_____

_____

_____

_____

Date	S M T W T F S	
Breakfast	Amount	Calories (kcal)
	Total	
Snack	Amount	Calories (kcal)
	Total	
Lunch	Amount	Calories (kcal)
	Total	

Snack	Amount	Calories (kcal)
	Total	
Dinner	Amount	Calories (kcal)
	Total	
Snack	Amount	Calories (kcal)
	Total	
Exercise	Duration	Calories burned (kcal)
Water									Fruit & Veggies								

Notes:

Don't rush the process, consistence delivers results!

Date:

Time	
6 am	
7	
8	
9	
10	
11	
12 pm	
1	
2	
3	
4	
5	
6	
7	
8	

Notes:_____

_____

_____

_____

To Do

Happiness

100%

75%   45%

60%

Accomplishments

☐. . . . .

☐. . . . .

☐. . . . .

☐. . . . .

Date	S M T W T F S	
Breakfast	Amount	Calories (kcal)
	Total	
Snack	Amount	Calories (kcal)
	Total	
Lunch	Amount	Calories (kcal)
	Total	

Snack	Amount	Calories (kcal)
	Total	
Dinner	Amount	Calories (kcal)
	Total	
Snack	Amount	Calories (kcal)
	Total	
Exercise	Duration	Calories burned (kcal)

Water										Fruit & Veggies							

Notes:

Don't let what you didn't do today get in the way of you can do tomorrow!

Date:

6 am	
7	
8	
9	
10	
11	
12 pm	
1	
2	
3	
4	
5	
6	
7	
8	

Notes:_____

_____

_____

_____

To Do

Happiness

100%

75%   45%

60%

Accomplishments

☐ . . . .

☐ . . . .

☐ . . . .

☐ . . . .

Date		S M T W T F S
Breakfast	Amount	Calories (kcal)
	Total	
Snack	Amount	Calories (kcal)
	Total	
Lunch	Amount	Calories (kcal)
	Total	

Snack	Amount	Calories (kcal)
	Total	
Dinner	Amount	Calories (kcal)
	Total	
Snack	Amount	Calories (kcal)
	Total	
Exercise	Duration	Calories burned (kcal)

Water								Fruit & Veggies								

Notes:

Don't rush the process, consistence delivers results!

Date:

Time	
6 am	
7	
8	
9	
10	
11	
12 pm	
1	
2	
3	
4	
5	
6	
7	
8	

Notes:_____

_____

_____

_____

To Do

Happiness

100%

75%   45%

60%

Accomplishments

☐ . . . .

☐ . . . .

☐ . . . .

☐ . . . .

Date	S M T W T F S	
Breakfast	Amount	Calories (kcal)
	Total	
Snack	Amount	Calories (kcal)
	Total	
Lunch	Amount	Calories (kcal)
	Total	

Snack	Amount	Calories (kcal)
	Total	
Dinner	Amount	Calories (kcal)
	Total	
Snack	Amount	Calories (kcal)
	Total	
Exercise	Duration	Calories burned (kcal)
Water									Fruit & Veggies							

Notes:

Don't let what you didn't do today get in the way of you can do tomorrow!

Date:

6 am
7
8
9
10
11
12 pm
1
2
3
4
5
6
7
8

Notes:_____

_____

_____

_____

To Do

Happiness

100%

75%   45%

60%

Accomplishments

☐ . . . .

☐ . . . .

☐ . . . .

☐ . . . .

Date		S M T W T F S	
Breakfast		Amount	Calories (kcal)
		Total	
Snack		Amount	Calories (kcal)
		Total	
Lunch		Amount	Calories (kcal)
		Total	

Snack	Amount	Calories (kcal)
	Total	
Dinner	Amount	Calories (kcal)
	Total	
Snack	Amount	Calories (kcal)
	Total	
Exercise	Duration	Calories burned (kcal)

Water									Fruit & Veggies							

Notes:

Don't rush the process, consistence delivers results!

Date:

6 am	
7	
8	
9	
10	
11	
12 pm	
1	
2	
3	
4	
5	
6	
7	
8	

To Do

Happiness

100%

75%   45%

60%

Accomplishments

☐ . . . .
☐ . . . .
☐ . . . .
☐ . . . .

Notes:_____

_____

_____

_____

Date		S M T W T F S
Breakfast	Amount	Calories (kcal)
	Total	
Snack	Amount	Calories (kcal)
	Total	
Lunch	Amount	Calories (kcal)
	Total	

Snack	Amount	Calories (kcal)
	Total	
Dinner	Amount	Calories (kcal)
	Total	
Snack	Amount	Calories (kcal)
	Total	
Exercise	Duration	Calories burned (kcal)
Water	Fruit & Veggies	

Notes:

Don't let what you didn't do today get in the way of you can do tomorrow!

Date:

6 am	
7	**To Do**
8	
9	
10	
11	
12 pm	
1	**Happiness**
2	
3	100%
4	75% 45%
5	
6	60%
7	**Accomplishments**
8	

Notes:_____

_____

_____

_____

Date		S M T W T F S
Breakfast	Amount	Calories (kcal)
	Total	
Snack	Amount	Calories (kcal)
	Total	
Lunch	Amount	Calories (kcal)
	Total	

Snack	Amount	Calories (kcal)
	Total	
Dinner	Amount	Calories (kcal)
	Total	
Snack	Amount	Calories (kcal)
	Total	
Exercise	Duration	Calories burned (kcal)
Water									Fruit & Veggies							

Notes:

Don't rush the process, consistence delivers results!

Date:

Time	
6 am	
7	
8	
9	
10	
11	
12 pm	
1	
2	
3	
4	
5	
6	
7	
8	

Notes:_____

_____

_____

_____

To Do

Happiness

100%

75% 45%

60%

Accomplishments

☐ . . . .

☐ . . . .

☐ . . . .

☐ . . . .

Date		S M T W T F S	
Breakfast	Amount	Calories (kcal)	
	Total		
Snack	Amount	Calories (kcal)	
	Total		
Lunch	Amount	Calories (kcal)	
	Total		

Snack	Amount	Calories (kcal)
	Total	
Dinner	Amount	Calories (kcal)
	Total	
Snack	Amount	Calories (kcal)
	Total	
Exercise	Duration	Calories burned (kcal)

Water								Fruit & Veggies							

Notes:

Don't let what you didn't do today get in the way of you can do tomorrow!

Date:

Time	
6 am	
7	
8	
9	
10	
11	
12 pm	
1	
2	
3	
4	
5	
6	
7	
8	

Notes:_____

_____

_____

_____

To Do

Happiness

100%

75%   45%

60%

Accomplishments

- ☐ . . . .
- ☐ . . . .
- ☐ . . . .
- ☐ . . . .

Date	S M T W T F S	
Breakfast	Amount	Calories (kcal)
	Total	
Snack	Amount	Calories (kcal)
	Total	
Lunch	Amount	Calories (kcal)
	Total	

Snack	Amount	Calories (kcal)
	Total	
Dinner	Amount	Calories (kcal)
	Total	
Snack	Amount	Calories (kcal)
	Total	
Exercise	Duration	Calories burned (kcal)
Water		Fruit & Veggies	

Notes:

Don't rush the process, consistence delivers results!

Date:

Time	
6 am	
7	
8	
9	
10	
11	
12 pm	
1	
2	
3	
4	
5	
6	
7	
8	

Notes: _____

_____

_____

_____

To Do

Happiness

100%

75%   45%

60%

Accomplishments

- [ ] . . . .
- [ ] . . . .
- [ ] . . . .
- [ ] . . . .

Date		S M T W T F S	
Breakfast		Amount	Calories (kcal)
		Total	
Snack		Amount	Calories (kcal)
		Total	
Lunch		Amount	Calories (kcal)
		Total	

Snack	Amount	Calories (kcal)
	Total	
Dinner	Amount	Calories (kcal)
	Total	
Snack	Amount	Calories (kcal)
	Total	
Exercise	Duration	Calories burned (kcal)

Water									Fruit & Veggies							

Notes:

Don't let what you didn't do today get in the way of you can do tomorrow!

6 am	
7	
8	
9	
10	
11	
12 pm	
1	
2	
3	
4	
5	
6	
7	
8	

To Do

Happiness

100%

75%   45%

60%

Accomplishments

☐ . . . .

☐ . . . .

☐ . . . .

☐ . . . .

Notes:_____

_____

_____

_____

Date		S M T W T F S
Breakfast	Amount	Calories (kcal)
	Total	
Snack	Amount	Calories (kcal)
	Total	
Lunch	Amount	Calories (kcal)
	Total	

Snack	Amount	Calories (kcal)
	Total	
Dinner	Amount	Calories (kcal)
	Total	
Snack	Amount	Calories (kcal)
	Total	
Exercise	Duration	Calories burned (kcal)
Water										Fruit & Veggies								

Notes:

Don't rush the process, consistence delivers results!

Date:

6 am	
7	
8	
9	
10	
11	
12 pm	
1	
2	
3	
4	
5	
6	
7	
8	

To Do

Happiness

100%

75%   45%

60%

Accomplishments

☐ . . . .
☐ . . . .
☐ . . . .
☐ . . . .

Notes:_____

_____

_____

_____

Date	S M T W T F S	
Breakfast	Amount	Calories (kcal)
	Total	
Snack	Amount	Calories (kcal)
	Total	
Lunch	Amount	Calories (kcal)
	Total	

Snack	Amount	Calories (kcal)
	Total	
Dinner	Amount	Calories (kcal)
	Total	
Snack	Amount	Calories (kcal)
	Total	
Exercise	Duration	Calories burned (kcal)

Water									Fruit & Veggies								

Notes:

Don't let what you didn't do today get in the way of you can do tomorrow!

Date:

6 am	
7	**To Do**
8	
9	
10	
11	
12 pm	
1	**Happiness**
2	
3	100%
4	75% 45%
5	60%
6	
7	**Accomplishments**
8	

Notes:_____

_____

_____

_____

Date		S M T W T F S
Breakfast	Amount	Calories (kcal)
	Total	
Snack	Amount	Calories (kcal)
	Total	
Lunch	Amount	Calories (kcal)
	Total	

Snack	Amount	Calories (kcal)
	Total	
Dinner	Amount	Calories (kcal)
	Total	
Snack	Amount	Calories (kcal)
	Total	
Exercise	Duration	Calories burned (kcal)

Water									Fruit & Veggies								

Notes:

Don't rush the process,
consistence delivers results!

Date:

6 am	
7	
8	
9	
10	
11	
12 pm	
1	
2	
3	
4	
5	
6	
7	
8	

To Do

Happiness

100%

75%   45%

60%

Accomplishments

☐ . . . .
☐ . . . .
☐ . . . .
☐ . . . .

Notes:_____

_____

_____

_____

Date		S M T W T F S	
Breakfast		Amount	Calories (kcal)
		Total	
Snack		Amount	Calories (kcal)
		Total	
Lunch		Amount	Calories (kcal)
		Total	

Snack	Amount	Calories (kcal)
	Total	
Dinner	Amount	Calories (kcal)
	Total	
Snack	Amount	Calories (kcal)
	Total	
Exercise	Duration	Calories burned (kcal)

Water									Fruit & Veggies								

Notes:

Don't let what you didn't do today get in the way of you can do tomorrow!

Date:

6 am

7

8

9

10

11

12 pm

1

2

3

4

5

6

7

8

Notes:_____

_____

_____

_____

To Do

Happiness

100%

75%   45%

60%

Accomplishments

☐ . . . .

☐ . . . .

☐ . . . .

☐ . . . .

Date		S M T W T F S	
Breakfast	Amount		Calories (kcal)
	Total		
Snack	Amount		Calories (kcal)
	Total		
Lunch	Amount		Calories (kcal)
	Total		

Snack	Amount	Calories (kcal)
	Total	
Dinner	Amount	Calories (kcal)
	Total	
Snack	Amount	Calories (kcal)
	Total	
Exercise	Duration	Calories burned (kcal)

Water									Fruit & Veggies							

Notes:

Don't rush the process, consistence delivers results!

Date:

Time	
6 am	
7	
8	
9	
10	
11	
12 pm	
1	
2	
3	
4	
5	
6	
7	
8	

Notes:_____

_____

_____

_____

To Do

Happiness

100%

75%   45%

60%

Accomplishments

☐ . . . .

☐ . . . .

☐ . . . .

☐ . . . .

Date		S M T W T F S
Breakfast	Amount	Calories (kcal)
	Total	
Snack	Amount	Calories (kcal)
	Total	
Lunch	Amount	Calories (kcal)
	Total	

Snack	Amount	Calories (kcal)
	Total	
Dinner	Amount	Calories (kcal)
	Total	
Snack	Amount	Calories (kcal)
	Total	
Exercise	Duration	Calories burned (kcal)

Water									Fruit & Veggies							

Notes:

Don't let what you didn't do today get in the way of you can do tomorrow!

Date:

6 am

7

8

9

10

11

12 pm

1

2

3

4

5

6

7

8

Notes:_____

_____

_____

_____

To Do

Happiness

100%

75% 45%

60%

Accomplishments

☐. . . . .

☐. . . . .

☐. . . . .

☐. . . . .

Date		S M T W T F S	
Breakfast		Amount	Calories (kcal)
		Total	
Snack		Amount	Calories (kcal)
		Total	
Lunch		Amount	Calories (kcal)
		Total	

Snack	Amount	Calories (kcal)
	Total	
Dinner	Amount	Calories (kcal)
	Total	
Snack	Amount	Calories (kcal)
	Total	
Exercise	Duration	Calories burned (kcal)

Water									Fruit & Veggies								

Notes:

Don't rush the process, consistence delivers results!

Date:

Time	
6 am	
7	
8	
9	
10	
11	
12 pm	
1	
2	
3	
4	
5	
6	
7	
8	

To Do

Happiness

100%

75%   45%

60%

Accomplishments

- ☐ . . . .
- ☐ . . . .
- ☐ . . . .
- ☐ . . . .

Notes: _____

_____

_____

_____

Date		S M T W T F S	
Breakfast		Amount	Calories (kcal)
		Total	
Snack		Amount	Calories (kcal)
		Total	
Lunch		Amount	Calories (kcal)
		Total	

Snack	Amount	Calories (kcal)
	Total	
Dinner	Amount	Calories (kcal)
	Total	
Snack	Amount	Calories (kcal)
	Total	
Exercise	Duration	Calories burned (kcal)
Water									**Fruit & Veggies**								

Notes:

Don't let what you didn't do today get in the way of you can do tomorrow!

Date:

6 am	
7	
8	
9	
10	
11	
12 pm	
1	
2	
3	
4	
5	
6	
7	
8	

To Do

Happiness

100%

75%   45%

60%

Accomplishments

☐ . . . .
☐ . . . .
☐ . . . .
☐ . . . .

Notes:_____

_____

_____

_____

Date	S M T W T F S	
Breakfast	Amount	Calories (kcal)
	Total	
Snack	Amount	Calories (kcal)
	Total	
Lunch	Amount	Calories (kcal)
	Total	

Snack	Amount	Calories (kcal)
	Total	
Dinner	Amount	Calories (kcal)
	Total	
Snack	Amount	Calories (kcal)
	Total	
Exercise	Duration	Calories burned (kcal)
Water									Fruit & Veggies								

Notes:

Don't rush the process, consistence delivers results!

Date:

6 am	
7	
8	
9	
10	
11	
12 pm	
1	
2	
3	
4	
5	
6	
7	
8	

To Do

Happiness

100%

75%   45%

60%

Accomplishments

☐ . . . .
☐ . . . .
☐ . . . .
☐ . . . .

Notes:_____

_____

_____

_____

Date		S M T W T F S	
Breakfast		Amount	Calories (kcal)
		Total	
Snack		Amount	Calories (kcal)
		Total	
Lunch		Amount	Calories (kcal)
		Total	

Snack	Amount	Calories (kcal)
	Total	
Dinner	Amount	Calories (kcal)
	Total	
Snack	Amount	Calories (kcal)
	Total	
Exercise	Duration	Calories burned (kcal)
Water		Fruit & Veggies	

Notes:

Don't let what you didn't do today get in the way of you can do tomorrow!

Date:

| 6 am |
| 7 |
| 8 |
| 9 |
| 10 |
| 11 |
| 12 pm |
| 1 |
| 2 |
| 3 |
| 4 |
| 5 |
| 6 |
| 7 |
| 8 |

Notes:_____
_____
_____
_____

To Do

Happiness

100%

75%   45%

60%

Accomplishments

☐ . . . .
☐ . . . .
☐ . . . .
☐ . . . .

Date	S M T W T F S	
Breakfast	Amount	Calories (kcal)
	Total	
Snack	Amount	Calories (kcal)
	Total	
Lunch	Amount	Calories (kcal)
	Total	

Snack	Amount	Calories (kcal)
	Total	
Dinner	Amount	Calories (kcal)
	Total	
Snack	Amount	Calories (kcal)
	Total	
Exercise	Duration	Calories burned (kcal)

Water									Fruit & Veggies								

Notes:

Don't rush the process, consistence delivers results!

Date:

Time	
6 am	
7	
8	
9	
10	
11	
12 pm	
1	
2	
3	
4	
5	
6	
7	
8	

To Do

Happiness

100%

75%   45%

60%

Accomplishments

☐ . . . .
☐ . . . .
☐ . . . .
☐ . . . .

Notes:_____

_____

_____

_____

Date	S M T W T F S	
Breakfast	Amount	Calories (kcal)
	Total	
Snack	Amount	Calories (kcal)
	Total	
Lunch	Amount	Calories (kcal)
	Total	

Snack	Amount	Calories (kcal)
	Total	
Dinner	Amount	Calories (kcal)
	Total	
Snack	Amount	Calories (kcal)
	Total	
Exercise	Duration	Calories burned (kcal)

Water									Fruit & Veggies								

Notes:

Don't let what you didn't do today get in the way of you can do tomorrow!

Date:

6 am	**To Do**
7	
8	
9	
10	
11	
12 pm	
1	**Happiness**
2	
3	100%
4	75% 45%
5	
6	60%
7	**Accomplishments**
8	

Notes:_____

_____

_____

_____

Date			S M T W T F S	
Breakfast		Amount		Calories (kcal)
		Total		
Snack		Amount		Calories (kcal)
		Total		
Lunch		Amount		Calories (kcal)
		Total		

Snack	Amount	Calories (kcal)
	Total	
Dinner	Amount	Calories (kcal)
	Total	
Snack	Amount	Calories (kcal)
	Total	
Exercise	Duration	Calories burned (kcal)
Water											Fruit & Veggies									

Notes:

Don't rush the process, consistence delivers results!

Date:

Time	
6 am	
7	
8	
9	
10	
11	
12 pm	
1	
2	
3	
4	
5	
6	
7	
8	

To Do

Happiness

100%

75%   45%

60%

Accomplishments

☐ . . . .

☐ . . . .

☐ . . . .

☐ . . . .

Notes:_____

_____

_____

_____

Date		S M T W T F S	
Breakfast		Amount	Calories (kcal)
		Total	
Snack		Amount	Calories (kcal)
		Total	
Lunch		Amount	Calories (kcal)
		Total	

Snack	Amount	Calories (kcal)
	Total	
Dinner	Amount	Calories (kcal)
	Total	
Snack	Amount	Calories (kcal)
	Total	
Exercise	Duration	Calories burned (kcal)

Water									Fruit & Veggies							

Notes: